Low Dose Naltrexone for Parkinson's Disease

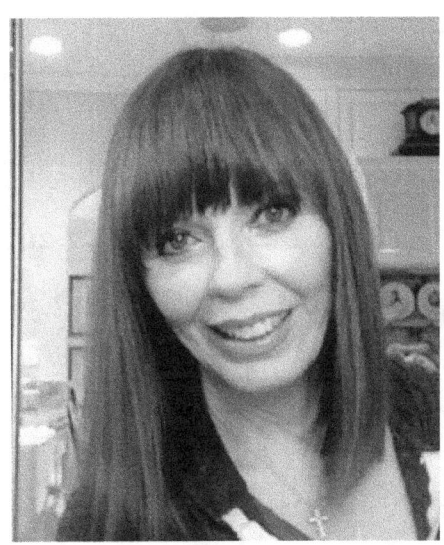

LOW DOSE NALTREXONE: LEXIE

© Parkinsons Recovery

Low Dose Naltrexone for Parkinson's Disease

Contents

LOW DOSE NALTREXONE: LEXIE 1

    What is Low Dose Naltrexone (LDN)? 11

    What website offers a lucid explanation of how LDN works in the body? 13

    Is a doctor's prescription necessary to obtain LDN? 14

    What's the best time of day to take LDN? 16

    Is LDN itself addictive? 16

    Can an individual take LDN with their other Parkinson's disease medications? . 18

    From your experience what would be a preferred dose of LDN to take? 19

    Can LDN be combined with painkillers? 20

    What diseases is LDN helpful for? 21

    How much does LDN cost? 21

    Are any clinical trials currently underway for LDN? 23

    What would you want to say to a person who has just been diagnosed with Parkinson's Disease? 24

    How to Hear Lexie on Parkinsons Recovery Radio 28

    About Lexie 28

© Parkinsons Recovery

Low Dose Naltrexone for Parkinson's Disease

LEXIE: I was officially diagnosed with Parkinson's disease in October of 2008. However, I had symptoms long before that, beginning about 20 years ago, when a very disturbing thing happened to me...I totally lost my sense of smell. In the beginning I had "smell hallucinations" and shortly after that my sense of smell was gone. Since other than my loss of smell, I felt fine, and I was extremely busy with my career, I didn't worry about it too much. Little did I know at the time that was my first actual "symptom" of PD.

They now know that losing one's sense of smell is a known pre-curser to the symptoms of Parkinson's disease and is a quite common complaint in those who are later diagnosed with PD. The loss of one's sense smell is really something to take seriously. If you do notice this in yourself or someone in your family, I would recommend that you see a Neurologist as soon as possible.

Shortly after I lost my sense of smell, I was having some problematic urinary incontinence which was very unusual for me since I'd never had children, so I consulted with a Urologist. He did some very extensive testing and found I had "bladder spasms". I asked him what could be the cause of my bladder spasms, which were quite severe. The doctor said that it could be one of two things, or it could

© Parkinsons Recovery

Low Dose Naltrexone for Parkinson's Disease

just be "idiopathic". I asked him what those two things might be and he said it could be either MS, or it could be Parkinson's disease. At the time, I had no known symptoms of Parkinson's disease, so that didn't even enter my mind. Then I got a little panicky thinking I might have MS, so I had an MRI for MS and nothing showed up in the test, so I was thrilled. The doctor said since I had no symptoms of PD and my MS MRI came back looking good, it was "idiopathic". I thought, "Well, if it's idiopathic than it is no big deal." Although I was a somewhat uncomfortable with the word "idiopathic" as I really don't believe anything that is this serious of a problem is "idiopathic" – to me "idiopathic" means "there is something wrong, but they don't know what it is". It was just easier for me to accept at the time that it was "idiopathic". Little did I know at the time, I had Parkinson's disease.

I also had a problem with insomnia that started about that same time my other two symptoms had surfaced. I'd never had a problem with sleeping and all of a sudden I had this terrible chronic insomnia and severe anxiety. I treated those symptoms with some of the new sleeping medications and an anti-depressant and just went along with my life and did the best I could.

© **Parkinsons Recovery**

Low Dose Naltrexone for Parkinson's Disease

In October of 2008, I remember I was sitting in the bathtub and I had one foot over the other and my right toe was tremoring and I thought, "What is this?" I called my husband in and I said, "Look at my toe...it is really shaking".

Shortly after that I was walking out in the yard and I was noticing that my right foot was not picking up; I was having a right foot drag. I was tripping and the only way I could describe the feeling was that it was like my brain wasn't telling my foot to lift up high enough when I was walking and I tripped and fell several times. I had to be very careful going up stairs because I was falling on the stairs. I also, at the same time, saw myself in the reflection of a large window in our house and noticed my right arm was not swinging naturally like my left arm was when I was walking. I thought that was odd. But it was my tripping and my right foot drag that caused me the real concern...this definitely was not normal.

I made an appointment with my Primary Care Physician and told him my story. He examined me and said that it might be Parkinson's disease and referred me to a Neurologist.

© Parkinsons Recovery

Low Dose Naltrexone for Parkinson's Disease

I went to a Neurologist, I actually consulted with three Neurologists – they did all of the standard tests and came to the same conclusion...I had Parkinson's Disease. Of course I was devastated. I will never forget the first Neurologist who diagnosed me and how I felt at the time and how "matter of factly" he gave me the bad news. I became very determined and my husband and I flew to Arizona to consult with the second Neurologist I saw at The Mayo Clinic in Scottsdale. Surely their Neurology Specialists would have a better answer for me, but to my disappointment, the diagnosis and the prognosis were the same.

What upset me the most was the "no hope" diagnosis....there was NO CURE for Parkinson's disease? All three had replied "no". I said, "Well, do you think that there would be a cure in my lifetime?" and, again, incredibly, all three looked at me and said "no". That, of course was the most devastating part for me because I am not the kind of person who can accept that kind of an answer. I have always been an optimistic, glass-is- half-full kind of person. My mom always used to tell me that I looked at the world through "rose colored lenses" and she was so right.

© Parkinsons Recovery

Low Dose Naltrexone for Parkinson's Disease

In the mean time my Parkinson's was progressing. I was having some severe issues with bradykinesia. It was like I was walking through quicksand or against the current of a river. That was one of my most debilitating symptoms. I had pain and stiffness, problems with my balance (I would bend over and if I didn't catch myself I would tip over onto the floor or hopefully into a wall). I also had this debilitating fatigue and a strange weak feeling in the back of my knees and legs, like the life was draining out of me. It really disturbed me when I started to have no motivation to do anything, which was a real problem because I had a very busy, high-pressure, high-stress job.

I found that I was losing my ability to handle stress – any kind of stress – especially work stress – I would just "short circuit" – things that used to be second nature to me – I could no longer do. I would look at my desk and just become "paralyzed" by all that I had to accomplish. This was definitely a problem. I had a dream job that I loved and I could no longer perform in the way that I used to. I was so concerned because I felt like I could no longer cope with anything that was in the least bit stressful. Life is filled with stress. My job was stressful. I have a Mom with Alzheimer's Disease and life is stressful. What was I going to do?

© Parkinsons Recovery

Low Dose Naltrexone for Parkinson's Disease

My usual confident voice was at times so shaky and soft that when I was talking to my clients on the phone or in person it was hard for me to disguise the fact that I had a problem.

I also had chronic and severe constipation, still had the urinary incontinence, which was now about as bad and embarrassing as it could possibly be, and most of the other non-motor symptoms that go along with Parkinson's disease. This is one of the reasons that many people call PD a "Boutique Disease", because there are cardinal symptoms that most people with PD have and then there are other symptoms that are unique to different individuals.

After consulting with the three Neurologists who were all Movement Disorder Specialists, this "rose-colored lens girl" finally concluded that Western Medicine was not going to cure my Parkinson's disease any time soon. That is when I started really looking at other alternative forms of medicine; something that would give me hope. All the neurologists could give me were "band-aid medications" that only masked my symptoms like the PD agonists. The agonist that I started on helped with my PD symptoms, but the side effects were a disaster for me.

© Parkinsons Recovery

Low Dose Naltrexone for Parkinson's Disease

One of the most serious side effects I had was falling asleep while driving. I did this four times in rush hour traffic before my Neurologist said "enough" and switched me to Carbidopa/Levadopa. It was only through the grace of God that I didn't kill myself or somebody else! Another side-effect I had on the Agonist was a compulsive shopping addiction.

I'm a woman and we all know that most women like to shop. I'm not a woman who really likes to shop. I am a destination shopper who shops when I need something, but I don't enjoy browsing around stores for hours on end. All of a sudden I developed the strangest shopping compulsion, not to shop at Nordstrom's (thank goodness!) but to shop at the Goodwill. I could not pass the Goodwill store that was about a mile from our house on my way home from work or any other time I got the chance. I just could not pass it without stopping in. It was like the steering wheel was just heading towards that Goodwill and I would spend an hour in there or longer until my husband would finally call me and ask me where I was. I got to the point where I was lying, I was telling him, "I'm at the grocery store." It was pretty severe, I thought, gosh, this is not normal, why do I feel the urgent need to shop at the Goodwill other than the fact that I was finding some

© Parkinsons Recovery

Low Dose Naltrexone for Parkinson's Disease

terrific bargains?! I was now even lying to my husband about where I was because he knew that I was shopping there every chance I got! I had become a shopping addict!

When I told my Neurologist about it and she kind of laughed because I was shopping at the Goodwill; at least I wasn't breaking the bank. But she said that was another reason the Agonists were not the right medication for me and that was when my medication was changed to the Carbidopa/Levadopa – another "band-aid" with fewer side effects for me.

I was now taking a 40 plus year old "gold standard" medication (!) that was helping with my symptoms, but in no way was helping with the progression of my disease. My doctor told me I could take it for about 5 years and I would feel great. I asked her "what would happen after 5 years" she then kind of looked away and didn't have much to say, but I knew. I had seen Michael J. Fox so many times on TV and in magazines – a true hero to me and so many others. Such a remarkable man who had PD for many more years than I did, and for all I knew he was only taking western medicine. I didn't want to go to the places he had to go, I didn't want to experience the same difficulties he was dealing with on a daily basis regarding his disease

© Parkinsons Recovery

Low Dose Naltrexone for Parkinson's Disease

after so many years of being on "band-aid" medications. The thought of not being able to tie my shoes terrified me.

I had to do something, so PD research became my part time job and it really paid off. I discovered Low Dose Naltrexone (LDN) about two and a half years ago and it has allowed me to titrate off of most all of my PD medications. Today, three years after my diagnosis, I don't look like I have Parkinson's disease and my symptoms are very, very minimal.

I have an occasional right hand and right foot and right arm tremor if I get really anxious or if I'm strenuously exercising. On occasion I get bradykinesia, but other than that, I'm just doing fantastic.

What is Low Dose Naltrexone (LDN)?

LEXIE: LDN has been a miracle for me. Low Dose Naltrexone *is a safe, inexpensive yet underused drug that's extremely beneficial with patients who have any condition marked by immune dysfunction. The great thing about this medication is that it has been used in much higher doses for decades to help people and patients recover from addiction to alcohol, heroin and other opiate drugs in high doses. Naltrexone by itself is a class of medications called*

Low Dose Naltrexone for Parkinson's Disease

antagonists; opium antagonists and in high doses of 50 to 100 milligrams, it works by decreasing the affects of opioid medications and street drugs. So it really had a very important function and it was FDA approved about 25 years ago in these very high doses.

However, in the 1980s, a New York City physician named <u>Bernard Bahari, MD</u>, discovered that very low doses of Naltrexone had profound effects on the immune system. So he began giving patients with AIDS 1.5 milligrams to 4.5 milligrams of Low Dose Naltrexone at bedtime and they had remarkable improvements. He then tried it with patients suffering with cancer and autoimmune disorders and he had equally good results.

Today LDN is recognized as a highly effective therapy for conditions ranging from cancer to autoimmune disorders to autism to Parkinson's disease to MS. There are so many diseases that it is helpful for. That's one of the great things about Low Dose Naltrexone. I have read reports about it helping with Lupus, rheumatoid arthritis, different cancers, chronic fatigue syndrome and of course, my success has been with Parkinson's disease.

© Parkinsons Recovery

Low Dose Naltrexone for Parkinson's Disease

> **What website offers a lucid explanation of how LDN works in the body?**

LEXIE: The website is www.ldnscience.org. You can watch a video on the first page that explains how LDN works in the body. LDN boosts levels of endorphins. We all know about endorphins. They are peptides that are produced in the brain and in the adrenal glands. They are best known for relieving pain and enhancing a sense of well-being. They're responsible for "runner's high" that is brought on by strenuous exercise. Runners get a rush of endorphins when they run.

These natural peptides are also powerful modulators of the immune system. When LDN is taken at bedtime, it actually attaches to the opioid receptors and temporarily blocks your own natural endorphins from producing. What this does is it signals the body to increase the production of endorphins because everything's been shut off for about 3 hours and the body goes, "Hey, what a minute. I don't have any endorphins here." So it helps to orchestrate the activity of stem cells, natural killer cells and other immune cells and as a result, LDN enhances the body's ability to fight disease. That's why it's so good for so many diseases.

People always say....How can one drug help so many

© Parkinsons Recovery

Low Dose Naltrexone for Parkinson's Disease

diseases?" It seems like an impossibility. The reason is that your immune system is being enhanced and your immune system is fighting disease.

Is a doctor's prescription necessary to obtain LDN?

LEXIE: Yes. You do need to get a prescription from your doctor. It is preferable that you get it through your Neurologist. However, I will say that it not an easy thing to do because the benefits of taking low doses of Naltrexone are not really known to our doctors and our Neurologists. Since it is a non-commercialized treatment doctors are never going to learn about it from drug company sales representatives. LDN is a generic drug. Many doctors are afraid of prescribing things off-label or doing something their colleagues don't do. The best chance of getting your doctor's cooperation is by showing them scientific basis for your requests like referring them to the www.ldnscience.org website. Bring in copies of some of the pages from the website and show them the studies that have been conducted to date. Sometimes that will convince your doctor that there is sufficient basis to prescribe LDN off-label.

Unfortunately it did not convince my Neurologist. I had a very well-known Neurologist in the city in which I live and

Low Dose Naltrexone for Parkinson's Disease

she just was very reluctant to prescribe it for me. It took me about four appointments to be able to get LDN. Finally, out of frustration, I cried and I said she was giving me no hope and I said, "I have to have hope. I can't just take "band-aid" medications…..what is going to happen to me in five years? What's going to happen to me in ten years?" She looked at me and she said, "You're right. You need hope." She researched LDN and the next morning she called me and she said she'd write a prescription for LDN for me. What she had done is she had actually contacted the manufacturers of one of the PD medications I was on and asked if it was okay for me to take LDN with their drug and the research department told her, yes, it was fine.

I thought it was interesting that the research department at this huge pharmaceutical company knew about Low Dose Naltrexone, but my doctor didn't. Then I agreed that " I would take LDN at my own risk" and the rest was history. After that, we had a much better relationship. She was no longer dreading my visits of pestering her about "partnering" with me on LDN – I really did want her to be a part of my experiment (progress!) I was now taking LDN with my Carbidopa/Levadopa and Azilect and every time I saw her, every three months, I was getting better and better. The only thing I could attribute that to was LDN.

© Parkinsons Recovery

Low Dose Naltrexone for Parkinson's Disease

She said I was having "a tremendous placebo effect," but I knew it was much more than a "placebo effect".

There are many people that I know who have Parkinson's disease that have asked their doctors a couple of times (or maybe more) for a prescription for LDN and their doctor keeps saying "no." The clincher for getting a prescription is to say that "You will take it at your own risk". They will write that down in your chart. When they know that you're taking it at your own risk, they feel less liable for something that they are not familiar with.

What's the best time of day to take LDN?

LEXIE: Through my experience, I have found that night time is the best time to take it. My own natural endorphins shut down while I am sleeping. However, LDN does sometimes disturb sleep in some individuals, so for these people taking it in the morning is preferred.

Is LDN itself addictive?

LEXIE: No. LDN is not addictive. However, when you stop taking LDN, it is possible that the symptoms of the disease may recur. I can give you an example of that. My husband and I were on vacation; we were gone for five days. Of all things, I forgot all my medications. At that time I had titrated my Carbidopa/Levadopa way, way back to almost

Low Dose Naltrexone for Parkinson's Disease

nothing, and of course I was off my PD Agonist. I was still on my Azilect (due to its neuroprotective benefits), but other than that, LDN was my primary treatment. We got down to this little resort town that happened to have a drug store. Lucky for me, it was the same chain drug store where I had all of my prescriptions refilled at home. We are about 6 hours from the town in which we live and I am thinking "Okay, I don't have my LDN.

Maybe what I can do is go into this pharmacy and at least get some Carbidopa/Levadopa, Azilect and some Xanax, which I hadn't taken since I started on LDN. Sure enough, they called my pharmacist and he told them to give me a five-day supply of the meds I requested. I could not get LDN because it is compounded medicine and there was certainly not a compounding pharmacy within several hundred miles of this resort town.

So I went away thinking, "Well I'm going to be okay for a few days". How wrong I was. I have to tell you, I was in very, very bad shape. I could not wait to get home. I was taking about 5 full 25/100 doses of Carbidopa/Levadopa a day. That was a huge amount for me since I had titrated down to almost none. I was also taking Xanax, because I was so anxious and I was taking my Azilect. It really ruined

Low Dose Naltrexone for Parkinson's Disease

my much anticipated trip because and I just could not wait to get home to get back on my LDN. On the fifth day we drove home and as soon as we arrived I took my LDN. The next morning, I was fine and I was just back to where I was prior to leaving for our trip.

So, it is possible to have a recurrence of your symptoms if you stop LDN for a certain length of time – for me it was 5 days. That is why LDN is a long term treatment. While it does not "cure" the disease it regulates the immune system's function and is helping to fight your disease. It's possible that some patients will experience what I did where they have a relapse when stopping it and others won't. But I happened to have a relapse and I'll tell you, I will never be without my LDN; forget my clothes, forget my cosmetics but not my LDN. Forget my husband, but not my LDN. Oh...he's not going to like that.

Can an individual take LDN with their other Parkinson's disease medications?

LEXIE: Yes, absolutely. It is absolutely recommended that you do because you need your Parkinson's disease medication until LDN has taken hold in your system enough where you can start very slowly titrating off your PD medications. Your own body will tell you when the time is

© Parkinsons Recovery

Low Dose Naltrexone for Parkinson's Disease

right to start titrating down your PD meds. When my "off times" became less and less was my signal that I may not need as much carbidopa/Levadopa as I had been taking. Every few weeks or so I would take ½ tab less, until I was totally titrated off.

The great thing about LDN is that most people get a sensation a couple of days after first starting on LDN – what most people report is a feeling of well-being (your body's natural endorphins!) I noticed this effect on about the second day. I just felt better. It was just like the lights went on. My brain wasn't as foggy and I just had this sense of well-being. It was a very hard thing to describe. I continued for about a year to take my LDN with my other PD medications before I slowly started titrating. Some people will be able to do this at a faster rate than I did. On the day that I was Carbidopa/Levadopa free I was thrilled. So yes, you do want to take LDN with your other PD medications and then just listen to your body. From my experience, you body will tell when it's time to very slowly start titrating off your PD meds.

From your experience what would be a preferred dose of LDN to take?

LEXIE: The average dose for most people is 4.5 milligrams.

© Parkinsons Recovery

Low Dose Naltrexone for Parkinson's Disease

That is what I'm taking right now. Some doctors start their patients off at 1.5 milligrams and then slowly go up to 2.5, 3 milligrams and then 4.5 which is basically the standard level. I have read where you can go up to ten milligrams of LDN. I don't know of anybody that's had to go up that high; 4.5 is generally the average dose. I started with 3 milligrams, which I did very well with. I'm doing absolutely fantastic on 4.5 milligrams and that is most likely where I will stay. Remember it is called Low Dose Naltrexone for a reason...low doses are what make it effective.

Since most doctors will not be familiar with LDN you will generally want to suggest to them, based on the literature, what the best dose would be. Be sure to bring in information from the www.ldnscience.org, which has a very helpful "question and answer section" you could print out for your doctor.

Can LDN be combined with painkillers?

LEXIE: No. LDN should never be combined with opiate or opiate-like painkillers, as it could neutralize their pain-killing effect for several hours. There is no reason why LDN cannot be combined with other types of painkillers such as NSAID's or Tylenol and other similar drugs.

© Parkinsons Recovery

Low Dose Naltrexone for Parkinson's Disease

What diseases is LDN helpful for?

LEXIE: What is so amazing – and this is what kind of threw me in the beginning – was that it is so beneficial for many diseases. I have seen reports about LDN benefiting diseases such as: ALS, Autism, Chron's Disease, Fibromyalgia, Lupus, Psoriasis, Alzheimer's Disease, Emphysema HIV-Aids, Multiple Sclerosis, Rheumatoid Arthritis, Colitis, Chronic Fatigue Syndrome, Inflammatory Bowel Disease and of course, Parkinson's Disease. I have also read about LDN benefiting (not curing) certain types of Cancer such as Bladder Cancer, Breast Cancer, Liver Cancer, Prostate Cancer, Colon Cancer, Lung Cancer, Ovarian Cancer just to name a few. So it's really a remarkable drug and so, so underused because our doctors just don't know about it.

How much does LDN cost?

LEXIE: Well that's the great news. We pay so much for our drugs. I remember when I was taking one of the Agonists in its non-generic form it was very, very expensive. I am still taking Azilect for its neuroprotective benefits and it is also very expensive. Fortunately my insurance company pays for 95% of it. The great thing about Low Dose Naltrexone is that the cost is about $39 a month because it is a generic drug.

© *Parkinsons Recovery*

Low Dose Naltrexone for Parkinson's Disease

LDN must be compounded at a compounding pharmacy, so you can't go to your local Walgreen's or Rite Aid; you will need to go to an actual compounding pharmacy. One thing that I would recommend is that you go to a compounding pharmacy that has compounded a lot of LDN. The reason I say that is I went to a compounding pharmacy near my home and they charged me $60 for my LDN. I asked them why it was so expensive. They answered that was the cost and that I was the only person they were compounding it for. Big red flag!! I took the LDN and I could feel that it wasn't working. So I took it back and I said, you know, there's something wrong with this LDN. I don't know what kind of filler you used or what it is, but it's not working. They took it back, they refunded my money and from then on I only get mine filled at compounding pharmacies that understand LDN and compound a lot of LDN prescriptions. I will give you a couple of names of compounding pharmacies that understand LDN:

    Custom Prescriptions in Bellevue, Washington. They compound a lot of LDN and you just give them your information. You can pay with a credit card and they will ship it to you.

    Skip's Pharmacy in Boca Rotan, Florida is a very big

© Parkinsons Recovery

Low Dose Naltrexone for Parkinson's Disease

advocate for LDN. People from all over the country get their LDN prescription from Skip's Pharmacy. Skip, the lead pharmacist, will actually speak to your Neurologist (if you can catch him) about LDN. Skip is such a big proponent of LDN. Again, you pay with a credit card and they will send it to your home.

So it's quite easy to get your prescription Rx filled, but you will most likely need to have it mailed to you, as I do, from Custom Pharmacy.

Are any clinical trials currently underway for LDN?

LEXIE: As of September 22 (2011) there is a petition that has gone to the White House and the Obama Administration to fund National Institutes of Health clinical trials of Low Dose Naltrexone for Multiple Sclerosis and that is a huge start. We need funding for clinical trials for LDN. Drug companies are not willing to fund LDN trials because this is a generic drug that has been around for many years. There simply is no incentive for them to do clinical trials. Yet, there are so many people, like myself, who are having phenomenal results with Low Dose Naltrexone. We need our doctors to know about LDN.

You can sign a petition supporting the LDN trial for MS by click on the following link and signing the petition:

© Parkinsons Recovery

Low Dose Naltrexone for Parkinson's Disease

http://wh.gov/gZa, It takes less than 5 minutes to sign the petition. It would really benefit all of us if you would visit the website and sign the petition even though the initial trial will be for MS patients. They don't ask for much information and the only thing that shows on the petition is your first name, your last initial and the city in which you live. We need to have these 5,000 signatures by October 22, 2011.

What would you want to say to a person who has just been diagnosed with Parkinson's Disease?

LEXIE: When you go to your Neurologist and they tell you there is no cure for Parkinson's disease – because that's the question that we all ask – please, please, please do not get discouraged. I was so depressed when I had three neurologists tell me that. I just decided somewhere in this world there is a treatment for Parkinson's disease. Somewhere in this world I'm going to get help and I'm going to get help for other people. That's when I started researching the internet and I found Low Dose Naltrexone. You're going to need to be on either one of the Agonists or Carbidopa/Levadopa. I would also ask your doctor right away for a prescription of LDN and would bring in information from the website www.ldnscience.org and tell them "I will take LDN at my own risk" along with your PD

© Parkinsons Recovery

Low Dose Naltrexone for Parkinson's Disease

medications. Please, just be persistent.

Your doctor will most likely say "no". Just don't take "no" for an answer. There's no reason why you should not be Low Dose Naltrexone right away – the earlier the better, but it works well even if you are many years into your disease as I have heard from many people who are taking it.

It is October of 2011 and I don't even have to tell people I have Parkinson's because nobody would know it. The only symptoms I have are occasional tremors I have when I'm over-exercising and a little bit of bradykinesia, but for the most part, I'm fine. One of the things that I did want to mention, if I'm going to be at a social function and I'm going to be "up" for a long, long time socializing, like at a wedding or something like that, every once in a while I will take a half a dose of Carbidopa/Levadopa just to make sure that I'm able to stay up. I don't know if I need it. I think I'm just using it as a crutch, but it's just something that I do. Maybe when I talk to you in six months I won't be doing that anymore, but, very occasionally, maybe once a week I take a half a dose of Carbidopa/Levadopa if I'm going to be planning for a very long day and evening.

Another thing that I would suggest is that there are some

© Parkinsons Recovery

Low Dose Naltrexone for Parkinson's Disease

issues I have found that many people with Parkinson's disease have in common. I would ask your doctor for tests on the following.

I would have your doctor do a blood test for your Vitamin B12 levels. Many people with Parkinson's disease are very low in B12. I was. I had to have injections Vitamin B 12 injections. Now I'm taking a sublingual form.

In the same blood test your doctor can check your Vitamin D 3 levels. Many people with Parkinson's disease are also low in this sunshine vitamin. I was extremely low and I take 5,000 IUs a day of Vitamin D3 just to keep my levels normal.

I would also recommend that you have a test done to see what your DHEA levels are. DHEA is your body's master hormone that regulates all of your other hormones. People with Parkinson's disease tend to be low in DHEA also. If you find out that you're low in any of these, your doctor will guide you how much supplementation you will need to take to bring your levels back to a normal state and you will feel much better.

Today, I feel like I don't even have Parkinson's disease, although I know that I do. I feel like I'm going to be able to lead a normal, long life like anybody else. I just never go

© Parkinsons Recovery

Low Dose Naltrexone for Parkinson's Disease

there in my head that I'm going to be disabled. It's so important to think positively and to know in your mind that you can get well.

I say it to everybody; "The body has the ability to heal itself if given what it needs," and that statement in itself is so encouraging to people. You don't have to get in the doldrums. You don't have to go down that road of seeing yourself disabled in the future. Just do everything that you can to get well knowing "That your body can heal itself if given what it needs to do so".

Exercise is a big part of your overall health – especially now. I never used to exercise. I had a busy career. I was naturally slender and I never exercised. I have to say I'm in the best shape of life now that I have Parkinson's Disease because I do Yoga and Pilates at the YMCA three times a week. I do 50 flights of stairs almost every day (it takes me about 15 minutes -I slowly worked up to 50 flights – I started with 5 flights, then 10 flights, etc.).

Please talk to your doctor about the amount of exercise that is best for you – just do whatever you can and do it every day. Even walking is a great exercise! I also eat a gluten-free diet. I have heard that many people with Parkinson's disease say they have intolerances to gluten,

Low Dose Naltrexone for Parkinson's Disease

so if you are having digestive issues you might want to just try eliminating gluten from your diet for one week and if it makes a difference, then consider yourself to be one of us, who is gluten intolerant.

How to Hear Lexie on Parkinsons Recovery Radio

Visit http://www.blogtalkradio.com/parkinsons-recovery and scroll back to find the show that aired October 5, 2011 featuring Lexie as my guest.

About Lexie

I'm a 63 year old woman. I live in the beautiful Pacific Northwest. I have been married for 16 years and while we have no children, we have lots of extended family and friends. As many of us, we do have a couple of adorable furry "kids" that are like "our children". I have had a professional career in the prestige cosmetic industry for the past 30 plus years; a career that I loved. While my work was high stress, it was a job that I truly enjoyed. I have been so blessed to have traveled to so many wonderful places and met some of the most amazing people during my career as an executive sales and training specialist. Unfortunately, I am no longer working because I have been diagnosed with Parkinson's Disease. I have now moved on to the next chapter of my life with

© *Parkinsons Recovery*

Low Dose Naltrexone for Parkinson's Disease

great hope for continued health, happiness and a heart for those I can support and encourage on their similar journeys, a journey that none of us asked for or expected...but here we are together in this place called "hope".

To order a DVD of Lexie's presentation at the Parkinsons Recovery Summit in Santa Fe visit:

www.summit.parkinsonsrecovery.com

www.ingramcontent.com/pod-product-compliance
Lightning Source LLC
Chambersburg PA
CBHW081756170526
45167CB00009B/4045